Table Of Contents

What Is The Ketogenic Diet

The Ketogenic diet (keto) is an eating plan that features a very low intake of carbohydrates, which are macronutrients found in food.

Low carb diets are eating plans that typically lower the intake of carbs to below 100 grams per day, the Ketogenic diet is the most strict of these and limits intake to less than 50 grams per day, preferably starting with 20 grams.

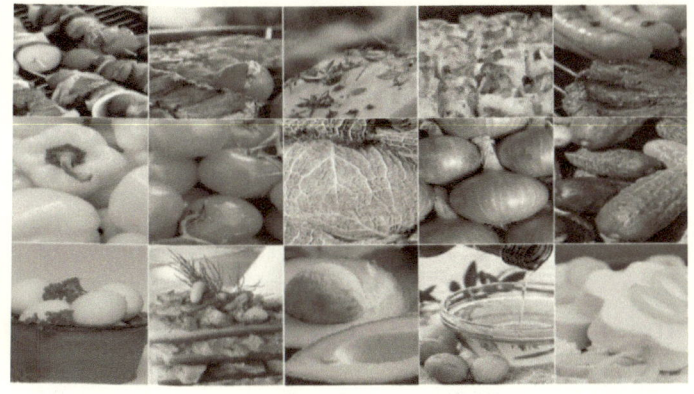

It is most important to understand that keto is not a fad diet, or a temporary solution to weight loss, it is actually designed to be a lifestyle plan that not only results in successful weight loss, but also promotes overall health, energy, and vitality.

It eliminates junk and processed food by definition, as most carbs are just that allowing you to eat clean, whole food for better overall health and wellness.

While some may question how sustainable it really is to drastically lower carb intake, in reality, it is quite easy with the wide variety of whole foods available, and several studies show they offer better results for weight loss than low fat diets, or even low calorie diets.

One of the reasons for this, besides various metabolic processes in the body, is that reducing carb intake naturally regulates the appetite, so people find they eat less naturally because they are satisfied and without starvation.

In general, a keto diet may be ideal for the overweight and obese, diabetics, anyone who needs to improve their metabolic health and for various other health reasons.

Types Of Ketogenic Diets

Keto is flexible and there are three distinct plans that target different goals.

Standard Ketogenic Diet (SKD)

This one is very low in carbs, with moderate protein, and high in healthy fats.

> ➢ *The ratio is typically, 75% fat, 20% protein and 5% carbs*

High-Protein Ketogenic Diet

This plan is similar to SKD, but incudes more protein.

> ➢ *The ratio is typically 60% fat, 35% protein and 5% carbs*

Cyclical Ketogenic Diet or CKD

This plan is widely used by athletes, bodybuilders, weight lifters and anyone participating in high intensity exercise and features short periods of high carb intake

> ➤ *5 keto days followed by 2 high carb intake days*

Targeted Ketogenic Diet or TKD

This plan is also used by bodybuilders, athletes and those who workout regularly to fuel intense workouts.

> ➤ *High load carb intake based around workouts*

Fuel Utilization In The Body: The Main Principle Of Keto

The body has three storage depots to use as fuel:

✓ Carbohydrates from food

✓ Protein that is converted to glucose in the liver and used for energy

✓ Stored body fat and ketones

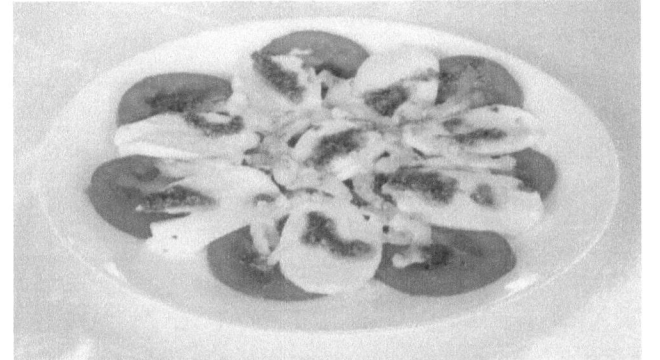

In a regular high carb diet, carbohydrates are the main source of fuel for the body.

1. Carbohydrates, *specifically starches and sugars* are readily broken down into glucose in the bloodstream, giving the body its principal energy source.

2. At this point, the hormone insulin steps in to remove glucose from the bloodstream as too much sugar can lead to a dangerous condition known as glycosylation.

3. Insulin converts glucose into glycogen. Some glycogen is stored inside the liver as a fuel reserve for the brain, and the rest is stored in the muscles as fuel reserves for the body.

4. When that muscle glycogen is not used through a lack of energy expenditure or exercise, it stays in the muscles.

5. The human body can only store so much glycogen, about 1800 calories worth. When that reserve becomes full both the muscles and the liver send a signal to stop insulin production and excess glucose from dietary carbs begins to build up in the bloodstream, calling for more and more insulin to be released to remove it.

6. Insulin levels surge, and eventually this leads to insulin resistance.

7. At this point, the liver then sends any excess glucose to be stored as body fat.

8. As high carb intake continues, glucose floods the bloodstream, insulin levels increase, and so do the body's fat stores. Eventually this leads to metabolic syndrome, a set of conditions caused by insulin resistance, which includes obesity, fatty liver, type 2 diabetes, heart disease, and other metabolic issues.

While this carb cycle may not occur in everyone, for many who are obese, have a sensitivity to carbs, or who do not expend the required amount of stored energy, this is often the case and the main culprit behind obesity.

Lipolysis And Ketosis

Under normal dietary conditions, ketones play no role in fueling the body and energy production, but during a Ketogenic low carb diet, ketones become the central player, fueling the body and at the same time flipping on the fat burning switch.

When the intake of carbs is limited, and their sources controlled, meaning that starches and sugars are eliminated, the body goes into a state called lipolysis, a most efficient biochemical pathway to weight loss and a scientifically proven alternative to using glucose for energy.

> ➤ Lipolysis is the only practical alternative to giving the body an alternative for glucose fuel, the process that often leads to obesity

> 1) Lipolysis occurs when the body begins to burn fat stores for energy instead of carbohydrates that are obtained from the diet.

2)   The by-products of this fat burning process are ketones and so ketosis is the secondary process of lipolysis.

3)   By lowering intake of carbohydrates and also the sources of those carbohydrates, which the body will use for energy first when available, it is forced to use its fat stores instead, literally melting it off the body in a state referred   to   as   ketosis.

> **Ketones, the byproduct of ketosis, fuel the body**

Sugars, grains, starches, and starchy vegetables fuel your body when you eat them, a state called glucosis (a term coined by the late Dr. Atkins, a pioneer in low carb weight loss). It is only when you lower carb intake and limit it to non-starchy vegetables, and small amounts of certain dairy foods that you are not eating enough carbs to create glucose, creating a state of ketosis where the body begins to burn its fat stores for energy.

➢ The only exception to the body not needing glucose for fuel is ketones

Lipolysis and its secondary process, ketosis provides adequate fuel for cells, the brain, and other organs just as glucose from carbs does BUT, unlike when the body uses glucose from carbs for energy, ketosis does not store fat, and actually allows the body to burn stored fat for fuel.

Ketosis Versus Ketoacidosis

Ketosis and ketoacidosis are often confused and they are two completely different things.

- Ketosis is a natural fat burning process in the body, while ketoacidosis is a medical condition that occurs only in uncontrolled diabetes.

- Ketoacidosis is dangerous, but ketosis on a ketogenic diet is perfectly normal, healthy, and necessary for weight loss.

Fuel Utilization By The Brain

According to Psychology Today, while the brain typically runs on glucose, it has no problems getting its fuel from ketones when they are available.

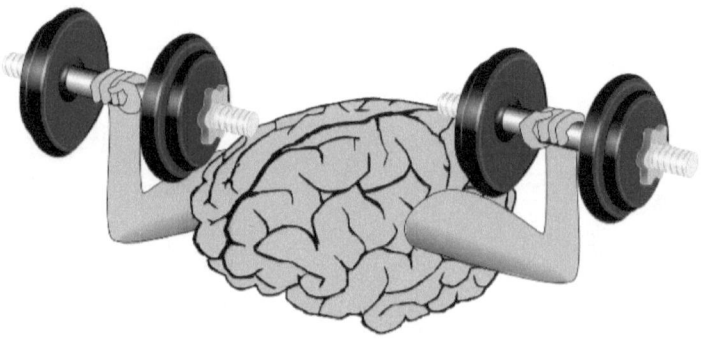

While some parts of the brain can only use glucose for energy, the body takes care of this too. When glucose is lacking, it can turn protein into glucose through a process called gluconeogenesis.

What The Science Shows

"Metabolic Effects of the Very-Low-Carbohydrate Diets" Findings

18

Findings published on the National Institutes Of Health website, Metabolic Effects of the Very-Low-Carbohydrate Diets: Misunderstood "Villains" of Human Metabolism, (Manninen et al) ascertains that reducing carb intake triggers a harmless physiological state known as ketosis, where ketones flow from the liver and spare the need for glucose metabolism providing an alternative source of fuel for the body.

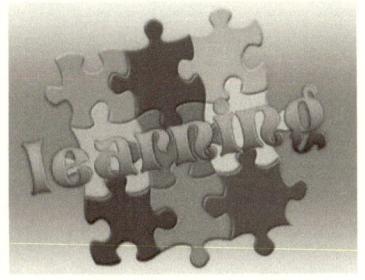

The report further states that there are *no clear requirements for dietary carbohydrates in human adults*, and that ketosis may offer therapeutic benefits for various different disease states, those common and also those that are rare.

The report further comments on **a landmark study that showed a very low carb diet results in significant reduction of body fat and a naturally accompanying increase in lean body mass in male subjects of normal body weight.**

Study From The American Journal of Clinical Nutrition

Ketogenic or low carb diets result in weight loss, as just one study conducted in 2008 and published in the American Journal of Clinical Nutrition reported a **12 pound weight loss in only 4 weeks in obese men who followed a low carb diet.**

Interestingly enough, all the studies' **subjects noted less hunger and more satisfaction on the low carb plan than while eating a low calorie diet.**

Stanford University Study

A study conducted at Stanford University (Christopher Gardner, et al) and funded by the National Center For Complementary and Integrative Health studied 311 overweight and obese pre-menopausal women and each one of the female subjects was randomly assigned one of four diets: Atkins™, Zone™, the LEARN™ diet or the Ornish™ diet.

Atkins was lowest in carbs, the Zone was low carb but higher in carbs than Atkins and the LEARN and Ornish diets were both regular carb but low fat plans.

The final results showed **the women on Atkins to lose the most weight**, an average of 10 pounds over 12 months and these women also **improved their metabolic profile**.

The Glycemic Index/GI Load Study

One study (Barclay AW, Petocz P, McMillan-Price J, et al. Glycemic index, glycemic load, and chronic disease risk–a meta-analysis of observational studies) concluded that **using the glycemic index** (GI scale that rates a food's ability to impact blood glucose levels) **to consume lower GI foods is associated with lower triglycerides and higher good HDL cholesterol lipid profiles.**

Duke University Medical Center Study

Another study conducted at Duke University Medical Center followed 120 obese subjects for six months. Half of the subjects followed the Atkins plan while the other half followed the American Heart Association's low-fat diet.

The **average loss for the Atkins group was 31 pounds, while the low fat diet averaged only a loss of 20 pounds.**

Atkins Diet Statistics

Atkins diet statistics published in 2003 in the distinguished New England Journal of Medicine reported **double the weight loss over a six-month period in those who followed Atkins, over those who followed a low-fat diet.**

The Mayo Clinic

The Mayo Clinic states that a **ketogenic diet may have desirable effects on diabetes, heart disease, and metabolic syndrome.** Additionally, **low carb eating is more effective at improving levels of bad LDL cholesterol** than moderate-carbohydrate diets.

Bayesian Analysis Of Weight Loss Dietary Therapy

The first ever conducted Bayesian study nf the effects of diet therapy on weight loss (Sackner-Bernstein, Kanter, Kaul), published in October of 2015 evaluated data from 17 randomized controlled trials of 1,797 people who were obese and overweight.

The evaluation **demonstrated more effective and greater weight loss and a reduced predictor of cardiovascular disease risk in those who followed a low carb diet versus a low fat diet.**

The Bayesian approach delivers insights, which are not always readily available in the traditionally used meta-analytical research and reveals the likelihood of a certain outcome in regards to the subject matter, a sort of summary that makes it easier for doctors to understand mass amounts of data.

These Findings Used The Following Parameters As To Diet And Study Subjects

Low-fat diet was based on a 30% or less of calories from fat diet

- The low carb diet was based on consumption of 120 grams or less of carbs per day

- All obese and overweight subjects did not have significant comorbidities

According to, Dr. Sackner-Bernstein, the leader of this Bayesian analysis, the results showed that a low carb diet had a 99% probability of resulting in greater weight loss.

Moreover, while there was a modest difference between the actual weight lost and health outcomes stemming from each diet, there was a **clear higher likelihood that reducing carb intake was superior to restricting fat.**

Saturated Fatty Acids and Risk of Coronary Heart Disease Study

Another study (Siri-Tarino, et al; Saturated Fatty Acids and Risk of Coronary Heart Disease) reported that **replacing saturated fat with refined carbs and sugars, something that has become commonplace in the United States in the last several decades is associated with either no improvement in or increased risks for cardiovascular disease as well as higher risks for dyslipidemia.**

The study's researchers advised that considering the current epidemic levels of insulin resistance as seen in the massive numbers of type 2 diabetes cases and obesity, **reducing intake of refined carbs and sugar along with weight control should be a top priority in the public's dietary goals.**

Benefits Of The Ketogenic Diet

WEIGHT LOSS

According to The CDC and the National Association Of Diabetes And Digestive And Kidney Diseases:

- ➢ More than 1/3 of the US adult population (35.7%) are obese

- ➢ More than 1 in 20 people, or 6.3% are extremely obese

- ➢ 74% of men (about 3 in 4 men) are either overweight or obese

- ➢ The incidence of obesity in both men and women is 36%

Many experts **attribute this epidemic in large part to a steady increase over time in the intake of unhealthy carbohydrate rich**

foods, including table sugar, simple sugars, sweets, refined starches and processed food.

According to one major statistical review (Cohen E, et al., Statistical Review of U.S. Macronutrient Consumption Data, 1965–2011), **the number of overweight and obese Americans rose from 42.3% to 66.1% from 1971 to 2011** <u>and</u> during this time:

➢ The consumption of *fat decreased* from **44.7% to 33.6%**

➢ The consumption of *carbohydrates increased* from **39%** to **50%** from 1965 to 2011

Experts, such as Dr. Sackner-Bernstein, surmise that statistics **imply a link between high carb intake in the American diet and obesity on a societal scale.** The analysis protocol of this study used data from various randomized clinical trials, which is the gold standard for assessing whether or not a particular treatment makes a real difference for any particular condition.

Low carb eating results in weight loss, and has done so for thousands of people who have struggled with their weight all of their lives.

Eating Low Carb:

✓ Eliminates those pesky out of control cravings

✓ Stabilizes blood sugar and consequently the appetite

✓ Research has shown that reducing carbohydrate consumption and replacing them with protein and healthy fats results in reducing overall calorie consumption naturally and without starvation.

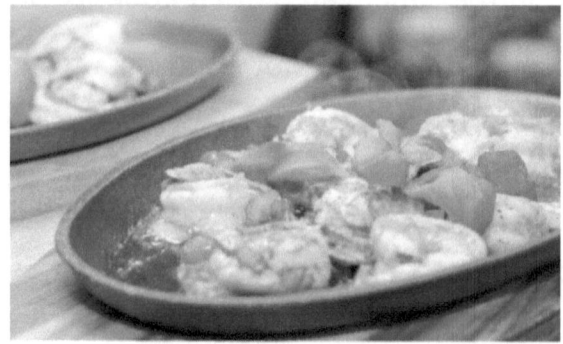

The side effects of weight loss and healthy weight maintenance are substantial, as obesity is linked to heart disease, type 2 diabetes, stroke, cancer, reduced quality of life, belly fat, joint problems, autoimmune disease, and premature death.

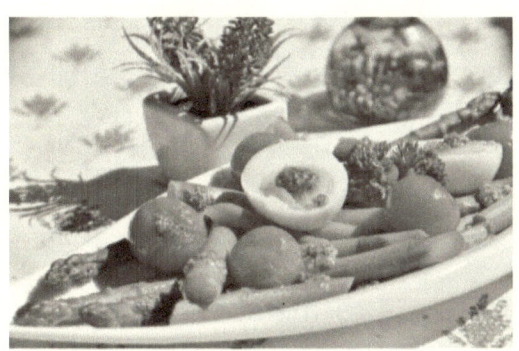

This is one of the main reasons that Keto is not a fad diet or a temporary solution; it is a lifestyle change that allows you to lose excess weight and maintain a healthy weight for ongoing health benefits.

STABILIZES BLOOD SUGARS

Since low carb eating eliminates insulin triggers, (sugars and starches) it is the diet of choice for those with prediabetes or those already diagnosed with type 1 or type 2 diabetes.

Eating a low carb diet reduces the need for the body to produce insulin, which is used to break down the glucose converted from diertay carbs in the blood stream.

High carb intake = high glucose = high insulin = high body fat

Reducing carb intake or insulin trigger foods, reduces the production of insulin in the body, and prevents the erratic blood sugar spikes that may lead to insulin resistance.

If this cycle continues, it eventually leads to metabolic syndrome, which is a set of conditions related to insulin resistance, and includes heart disease, obesity, fatty liver, and type 2 diabetes.

Of course, anyone who is considering changes to their diet should consult their doctor. This is particularly the case if you are taking medication for your diabetes, as this may need to be adjusted too.

LOWER LEVELS OF VISCERAL FAT

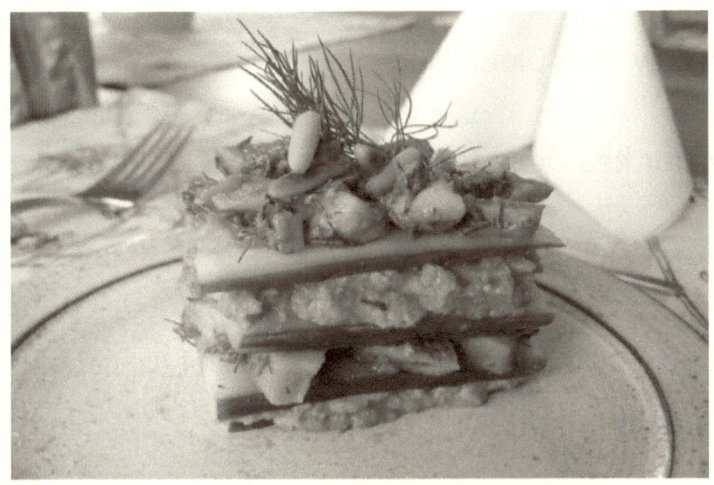

Research has shown that a low carb diet can help to reduce levels of visceral fat specifically rather than the superficial subcutaneous fat.

Visceral fat or belly fat is the most dangerous type of fat that is deeply embedded around major organs inside the body and a recent large study showed a significant correlation between waist size and reduced life expectancy in both men and women.

MAINTAIN HEALTHY BLOOD PRESSURE

High blood pressure poses serious risks for heart disease and stroke. A low carb diet may help to maintain healthy blood pressure.Other Benefits Or Uses Of A Low Carb Diet Include...

✓ May lower risks for heart disease, diabetes, cancer, and stroke

✓ May lower risks for gallbladder disease

✓ The ketogenic diet is used to treat several types of cancer and to slow the growth of tumors

✓ The ketogenic diet is also used to treat traumatic brain injury, epilepsy, Parkinson's disease, Alzheimer's disease and polycystic ovary syndrome

How Reducing Carb Intake Affects Appetite

One of the most amazing effects of the Keto diet or any significant reduction of carb intake is how it significantly changes the appetite.

✓ Hunger is reduced

✓ Out of control cravings for sugar, sweets and other carbs are gone

✓ Many report they no longer wake up in the middle of the night to sleep eat, a common occurrence among those whose appetite is wrecked by carbs

✓ Calorie counting becomes obsolete as the appetite is reduced naturally and low carb eaters simply want and need less food, without starvation or will power. This is the reason why Keto does not include calorie counting, but instead advises people to eat to satisfaction, which amazingly comes from much less food than when carb intake is substantial.

Why is this so? There are two main reasons.

The Leptin Equation

The hunger-regulating hormone leptin works in the brain to send signals to the body that you are full, so it registers the need to decrease food consumption, increase metabolic rate and shut off the hunger response. This is a complicated process, and an ongoing cycle that repeats itself, as you get hungry again and again throughout the day.

Therefore, as the levels of leptin rise and wane, so does the sense of hunger (up or down) and to some extent your metabolic rate.

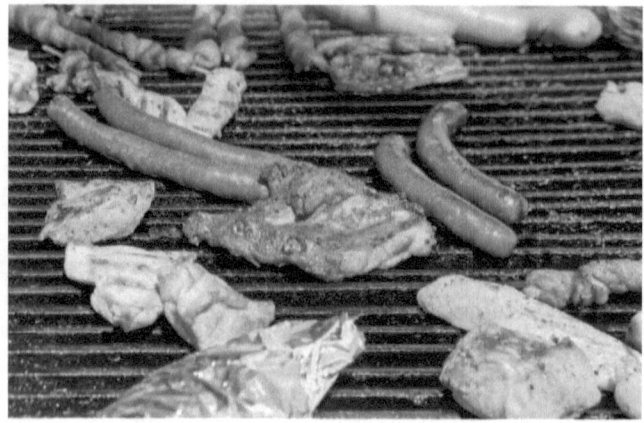

Between meals, your fat mass decreases in size as it is being used for energy, and so does the level of leptin. Less leptin crosses the blood brain barrier, less binds to its receptors and the brain sends the signal to let you know it's time to eat again.

The critical point is **when leptin crosses the BBB, because if it cannot make it across, the hunger response is never shut off, no matter how much leptin there maybe in the blood stream**.

This problem, and the often the plight of the obese is when leptin never reaches their brain to shut-off the hunger response, and hunger results in eating, which more makes more fat stores, which makes more leptin, which cannot shut off the hunger response because it cannot get to the brain, in a never ending cycle.

Why does this happen?

Researches from St. Louis and Japan (Banks A, Coon AB, Robinson SM, Moinuddin A, Shultz JM, Nakaoke R, Morley JE, et all, Triglycerides induce leptin resistance at the blood-brain barrier) figured out that **triglycerides, which are fats found in the blood stream interrupt the passage of leptin across the blood brain barrier.**

When triglyceride levels are high, as they are in most overweight and obese people, they block this passage of leptin where it can signal that the body has had enough food and is satisfied.

What does this have to do with a low carb diet?

It is a well-known fact that a **low-carb diet results in a dramatic reduction in triglyceride levels. This reduction ensures that leptin can get to the brain to successfully reduce hunger.**

The **reduction in triglycerides happens pretty fast once carb intake is reduced, and is one of the main reasons that low carb eaters have a substantial reduction in hunger.** As an added benefit, once leptin gets to the brain it boosts thermogenesis (fat burning) and so the metabolic rate increases.

This is also one of the main reasons that low-carb wins the battle over low fat diet plans. A low carb diet can result in a naturally lower caloric intake as people are simply not as hungry as they are when eating many carbs.

They are not white knuckling it through caloric restrictions as they do on the many high carb/low fat plans where people need much more support to get through the dietary day.

Conversely, low fat diets raise triglycerides levels and eventually most who follow these types of plans will give into that hunger.

Blood Insulin Levels

Another way that limiting carbs regulates appetite is by regulating insulin. Researchers at Temple University School of Medicine found that **lowering carb intake alters blood insulin levels in ways to promote appetite suppression and satiety.**

10 obese people with type 2 diabetes were placed in the hospital 14 days, and each bite of food they took was analyzed and daily blood samples were taken. For 7 days they ate a normal diet, then for 14 days, their carb intake was limited to 21 grams per day, and they were allowed to east as much protein and fat as they wanted.

➢ In the end, analysis showed they ate 1/3 fewer calories on the low carb days, than they ate on the 14 days of a regular diet that included carbs

➢ They lost an average of 3.5 pounds during the low carb days

➢ Their blood insulin levels dropped by 23%, which resulted in the suppression of appetite

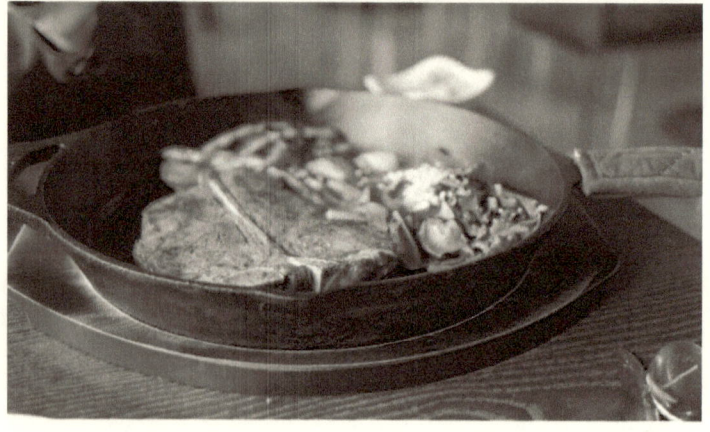

Carbohydrates stimulate the appetite and also cause out of control **cravings**, in part due to the erratic blood sugar swings and insulin hikes they cause, but a **low carb diet** actually works as natural appetite suppressant.

This is one of the main reasons that keto and other low carb plans work very well for those who have struggled all their lives white knuckling it through the various low calorie and low fat diets they have endured.

In many cases, there is no willpower, hunger is not an issue, and a new lifestyle takes over naturally.

A Closer Look At Carbohydrates

Carbohydrates are one of the three main macronutrients; the others are protein and fat.

Carbohydrates are biomolecules or saccharides, in simple terms, carbohydrates are sugars. In order to understand how the Ketogenic diet works, it is important to understand carbohydrates and what they do inside the body.

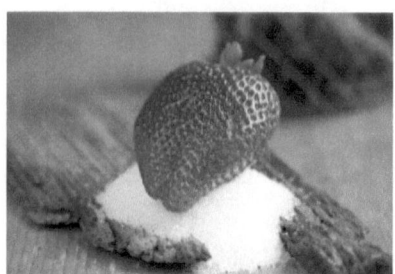

Types Of Carbohydrates

There are two types of carbs, traditionally classified as simple and complex.

Simple Carbohydrates

Simple carbs are those made from only one or two sugar (saccharide) chains. All simple sugars and starches are converted to glucose in the body, except sugar alcohols and insoluble fiber.

Types Of Simple Sugars

- Sucrose is table sugar or cane sugar and all items made with it

- Glucose is found in some fruits and starchy vegetables

- Fructose is the sugar in all fruits and honey and is also used to make many processed food products because of its high level of sweetness

- Galactose is the sugar that occurs naturally in dairy, like milk and yogurt

Naturally occurring sugars are those found naturally in a food or in the ingredients used to make a food, for example fruit, milk and vegetables.

Added sugars refer to those added during cooking or manufacturing, and include, corn syrup, honey, or table sugar. Table sugar and many things made with it are considered to be an empty calorie food that serves absolutely no nutritional benefits in the body.

Simple Carbohydrates Include: non-starchy vegetables, candy, table sugar and anything made from it, soda, white flour, juices, fruit, milk, honey and syrup just to name a few.

With the exception of non-starchy vegetable, **simple carbs require no break down as they enter the body to be absorbed so they digest** quickly to flood the bloodstream with glucose, causing insulin spikes to occur.

This process **triggers the release of insulin** from the pancreas, which sends food to cells, and any leftover sugar is stored as fat, which **contributes to weight gain and obesity.**

The constant stimulation of the production of insulin may and does at epidemic levels in the United States, **eventually lead to insulin resistance, a condition known as type 2 diabetes.**

Complex Carbohydrates

Complex carbs are made up of thousands of sugar chains hence the name complex.

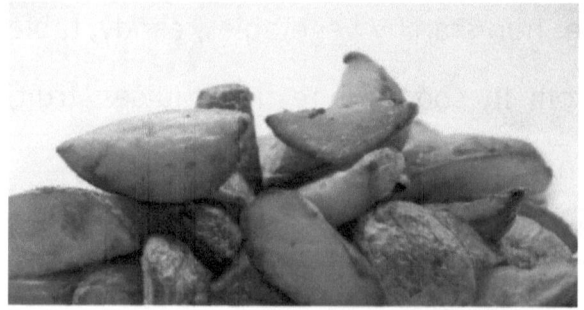

Complex Carbohydrates: any starch including but not limited to corn, potatoes, beans, rice, grains, cereals, and bread.

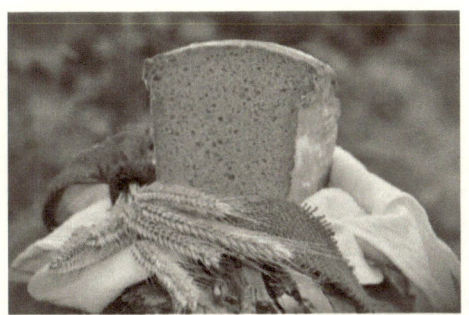

While some may argue that complex carbs are "better" than simple carbs, low carb diets, like the **Ketogenic take a different viewpoint, which is that both simple and complex carbs are insulin triggers** that provide the body with a fuel source that can turn to stored fat (glucose).

Glycemic Load

Doctors and other researchers in the Harvard Nurses Health Study found that **baked potatoes and cold cereal were foods that contributed most to increasing blood sugar levels to an unacceptable level,** known as "glycemic load."

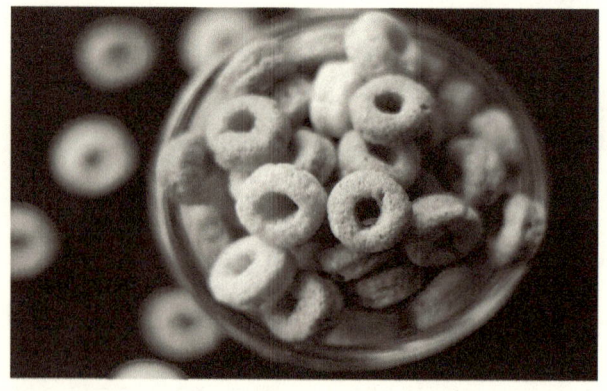

The Nurses' Health Study both part 1 and part 2 is the largest epidemiological study conducted in the US into the risk factors for major chronic diseases in women and has been going strong since 1976. 75,521 women aged 38 to 63 who had no previous diagnosis of diabetes, angina, myocardial infarction, stroke, or any other cardiovascular conditions were followed for ten years (Liu, S., Willett, W.C., Stampfer, M.J., et al).

During the 10 year follow up, the study documented 761 cases of coronary heart disease, 208 of which were fatal and 553 nonfatal, and **dietary glycemic load was directly associated with risk of cardiovascular heart disease** even when adjustments for smoking status, age, and total caloric intake and other risk factors for heart disease were accounted for.

The Glycemic Index

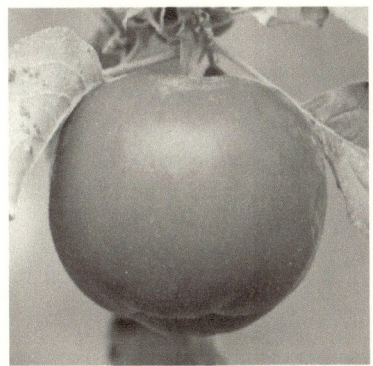

The Glycemic Index (GI) is a scale of 1 to 100 that measures a food's impact on raising blood sugars or its glycemic load. The higher the score a food has the higher the glycemic load.

Simple Versus Complex Carb on the GI Scale

> A white potato without skin has a GI of 98, while one raw apple has a 34 GI

The potato is considered a complex carb, while the apple is considered to be a simple carb.

Any foods that are considered to cause significant insulin release will typically be high on the GI scale.

Carbs And Ketosis

All carbs, both simple and complex convert to glucose in the body, which is then used as fuel and energy for cells and other organs inside the body.

Sugar Alcohols

In general, sugar alcohols are not insulin triggers and they do not count as impact carbs, but some do have a higher GI than others and should be considered carefully and monitored for their effect on your individual results.

Individual results can vary as to the digestion of sugar alcohols depending upon an individual's gut enzymes and how the sweeteners are consumed.

Sugar Alcohol	Glycemic Index
Maltitol	36
Xylitol	13
Sorbitol	9
Glycerol	3
Isomalt	2
Mannitol	0
Erythritol	0

Reducing Carbs To Induce Ketosis

The use of carbs for fuel is exactly what the ketogenic diet aims to avoid by greatly limiting carbs and their sources in order to give the body its alternative energy source, which is fat.

> ➢ The main source of carbohydrates in the Ketogenic diet is non-starchy vegetables

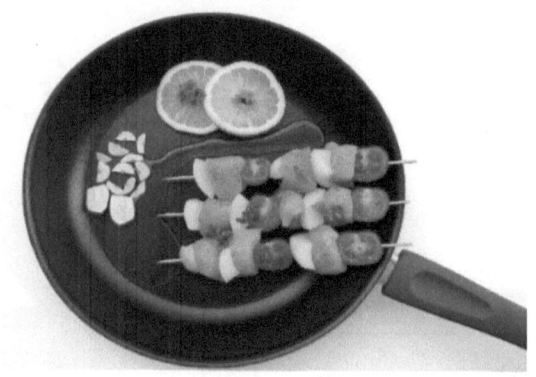

This is especially **strict in the beginning weeks in order to trigger ketosis**.

But wait, aren't vegetables simple carbs? Yes, they are but...

➢ Non-starchy vegetables are not insulin triggers

➢ Non-starchy vegetables are very low in carbs, making them a nutrient dense food with a very low glycemic load that supports ketosis

The following carbs are not allowed...

- Sugar or foods made with it
- Fruit
- Rice
- Pasta
- Bread
- Milk
- Starchy vegetables
- Any other starches

➢ The Ketogenic diet advises less than 20 grams of net carbs per day, most of which should come from non-starchy vegetables.

How To Calculate Impact Carbs

The Role Of Fiber

Fiber is naturally found in many carbohydrates, and remember fiber does not turn into glucose in the body as other sugar carbs do, and so that fiber helps to lower the glycemic load of carb rich foods.

Net Carb Formula

The **Ketogenic diet only counts what are known as Net Carbs** and the formula to figure out the net carbs of any food is simple.

The more fiber a food has, the less impact its carbohydrates will have on blood sugars.

THE NET CARB FORMULA

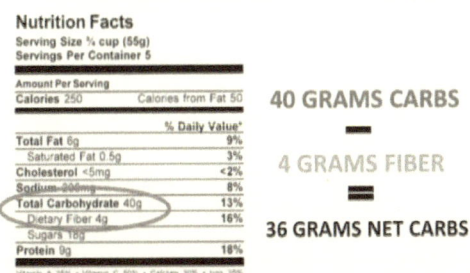

40 GRAMS CARBS

—

4 GRAMS FIBER

=

36 GRAMS NET CARBS

This formula makes it easy to determine the actual impact carbs of any food by simply reading the food labels or looking at its nutritional value.

Key Considerations For Fiber And Carbs

✓ **Fiber does not negate carbs**, it just lowers the impact of carbs that naturally occur within that food. For example, an avocado has 17 grams of carbs, and 13 grams of fiber, yielding 4 grams of net carbs. 1 cup of ice cream has 32 grams of carbs, but mashing in an avocado to that ice cream will not reduce it by the 13 grams of fiber in the avocado

✓ Sugar count listed in the carbohydrates section of a food label is exactly that, sugar. Typically this means the label has separated sugar and fiber in the total carb count

✓ **No credible evidence exists as to the effectiveness of so called "carb blockers"** or supplements that claim to slow the absorption of carbohydrates

✓ **There is no such thing as negative carbs,** this happens with incorrect calculations and in some food tracking apps when fiber is subtracted from a food that has listed starches and sugars separately from fiber

Rules Of The Ketogenic Diet

CARB INTAKE → Less **than 50 grams of net carbs per day,** but **better at 20 grams** at least in the beginning

✓ Most of the carbs should come from non-starchy vegetables

✓ Green, fibrous vegetables are your best choices, though many other low carb vegetables are fine

✓ Always eat a carb food with a protein or a fat, for example have a piece of cheese with cucumbers or salad with chicken.

LOTS OF HEALTHY FATS → Don't be afraid of fats. Fat is 90% ketogenic. Remember that in ketosis, fat is the main energy source for the body, helps remove hunger, provides key macronutrient requirements and natural fats are fine when controlling carb intake. They also have many other benefits, including providing the building blocks for several important hormones and bodily structures.

✓ The best fats are monounsaturated and saturated, including olive oil, grass fed butter, red meat, and coconut oil. Margarine is never advised, as it is fake and interferes with ketosis. Natural whole fats are always best.

✓ Limit intake of polyunsaturated fats, including soybean oil, corn oil, and cottonseed oil.

✓ Fat intake is variable and depends on weight loss goals.

ADEQUATE PROTEIN → Protein is both 46% ketogenic and 58% anti-ketogenic, as some protein will convert to glucose in the bloodstream and inhibit ketosis, so intake should be enough to prevent muscle loss, but not so much that will disrupt ketosis.

Protein Intake Guidelines

> ➢ **Sedentary lifestyle:** 0.69 - 0.8 grams per pound of lean body mass

> ➢ **Mildly active:** 0.8 to 1 gram per pound of lean body mass

> ➢ **Heavy strength training/bodybuilding and exercise:** 1 to 1.2 grams per pound of lean body mass

Lean body mass is typically defined as - *body weight minus body fat*

- Men will have a higher lean body mass than women, and typically, it is 60% to 90% of the total body mass.

- You can use any of a number of online lean body mass calculators, such as this one - http://www.calculator.net/lean-body-mass-calculator.html to figure yours.

- If you use a Fat Caliper to measure your exact body fat, than you will get a much more accurate lean body mass index measurement.

- Keep in mind these protein intake recommendations are just general guidelines.

Protein Choices

- ✓ Fatty red meats, chicken with skin, turkey, eggs, deli meats, seafood and fish

- ✓ Nuts, seeds and full fat dairy such as heavy cream and sour cream should be taken in moderation as these protein sources are higher in carbs than meat, fish or poultry which have zero carbs

EAT TO SATISFACTION → Eat when hungry until you feel satisfied

INCREASE SALT INTAKE → A little extra salt, can help avoid possible side effects known as keto flu as your body adjusts to ketosis, including headaches, muscle cramps or weakness that occur as result of an electrolyte imbalance and since a low carb diet is naturally diuretic, you don't have to avoid salt to minimize water retention.

- ✓ Get that salt from 1 to 2 cups of broth daily or soy sauce over food

Caution: ask your doctor about increasing salt, and if you are being treated for a condition that requires limited sodium intake, like hypertension continue with the medical advice of your doctor.

DRINK LOTS OF WATER → Water is a natural appetite suppressant and also supports the body's ability to metabolize fat. Several studies found that reducing intake of water may cause fat deposits to increase, while drinking more reduces them.

Hydration greatly promotes weight loss, so drink lots of fresh water throughout the day. The more active you are the more hydration you will need.

Evaluating Macronutrients In Ketosis

Carbohydrate, protein, and fat are all macronutrients that have differing effects on ketosis based on how they are digested and how each affects glucose levels in the blood.

- ✓ Carbohydrates are 100% anti-ketogenic due to their ability to raise both glucose and insulin levels in the blood

- ✓ Protein is 46% ketogenic and 58% anti-ketogenic because more than 50% of all protein from food is converted to glucose that raises insulin

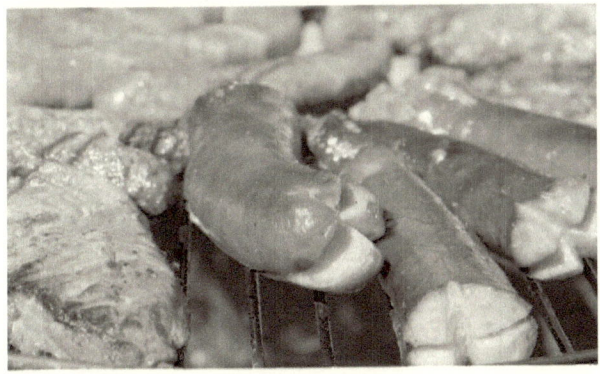

- ✓ Fat is 90% ketogenic and only 10% anti-ketogenic representing the conversion of the glycerol portion of triglycerides to glucose. Eating fats has minimal effect on ketosis in the literal sense; it is more of an effect on how much body fat versus dietary fat is burned as fuel in the body.

When in Doubt, Eat Less Carbs and More Fat

Choosing The Right Fats In Keto

Contrary to all the hype about fat, replacing sugar and carbs with healthy fats actually does result in weight loss, as shown by many studies.

It also true that **low-carb diets have been shown to result in more weight loss and a larger reduction in cholesterol levels than low fat diets.**

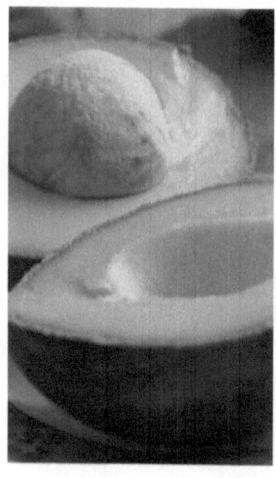

Fat does not make you fat in it of itself, fat has more calories than carbs or protein, so a high intake of fat may result in a higher caloric intake, which can cause weight gain under normal dietary conditions.

Additionally, it is when carbs and fat are mixed that problems in weight gain arise. The only proof you really need to this fact is the insurmountable amount of carb/fat laden junk food and processed food that we consume as a society that in great part has resulted in the epidemic levels of obesity (1/3 of all US adults) in the United States.

When you limit carb intake, the body will use dietary fats and your own fat stores for energy, literally turning your body into a fat burning machine, helping to reduce belly, thigh, and hip fat.

What Fat Does Inside The Body

While fat has more calories, 9 per gram versus the 4 per gram in both protein and carbs, it's more important to understand what it does inside the body.

When you are young your metabolism and high activity levels may allow you to eat carbs and fats and maintain a healthy weight, but as you get older and activity levels and metabolism slow down the weight may start to creep up.

If you are already overweight and your diet is filled with carbs, it makes it very difficult for the body to use stored fat for energy because it always defaults to carbs for that purpose.

✓ Greatly reducing carb intake promotes the body's ability to burn fat stores for energy resulting in healthy weight loss.

✓ Unlike carbs, fat also promotes satiety and fullness, helping to regulate the appetite so you actually eat less. In fact, you have to eat two times more carb calories as fat calories to reach the same level of fullness.

✓ Unlike carbs, fat has little impact on blood glucose, which keeps blood sugars stable, eliminating out of control cravings and hunger that comes after eating carbs.

Types Of Fats

✓ Monounsaturated fats are found in avocados, nuts, olive oil and canola oil,

✓ Polyunsaturated fats are found in vegetable, seed and nut oils, like soybean, corn and sesame oils along with fatty fish like salmon and sardines.

✓ Essential fatty acids include both omega-3 and omega-6 fatty acids that the body cannot produce on its own. Shellfish is rich in omega-3s and you can get omega-6s from chicken, pork, and seeds.

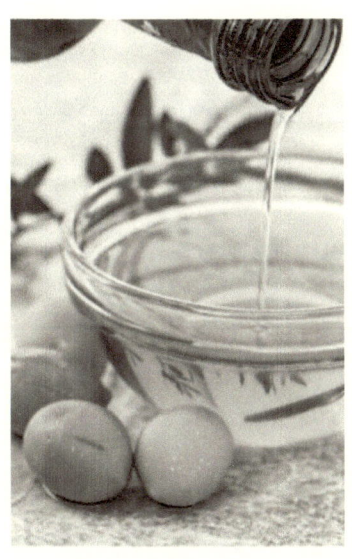

✓ Ideally, you need to balance intake of both omega-3s and omega 6 fatty acids with a balanced combination of shellfish, fatty fish and nuts, canola oil and flaxseed.

✓ Saturated fats are those that are solid at room temperature, and their best sources on a low carb diet are butter, red meat, and coconut oil. Since the target of the Ketogenic diet is to burn fat for energy consuming these types of fats is not only acceptable, but also required, and many studies confirm that this fat intake while on a low carb diet does not raise cholesterol or fat levels in the blood.

✓ Trans fats (also known as partially hydrogenated vegetable oil or hydrogenated vegetable oil) are bad news, increase risk for heart disease and should always be avoided when eating a Keto diet. These are typically found in fried foods, sweets, baked goods, processed snacks and food products, cookies, crackers and vegetable shortenings.

Optimal Fat Intake

Remember, the goal of fat is to provide satiety, boost energy, increase metabolism and support the enjoyment of food as fats make everything taste better.

It is not advisable to eat so much fat that you send your caloric intake through the roof. The following guidelines can help you get an idea of daily fat intake; of course, body size will determine the portions, as larger men will eat more than smaller women will. You can choose fats in any combinations you see fit.

Daily Fat Intake Guidelines:

Seafood

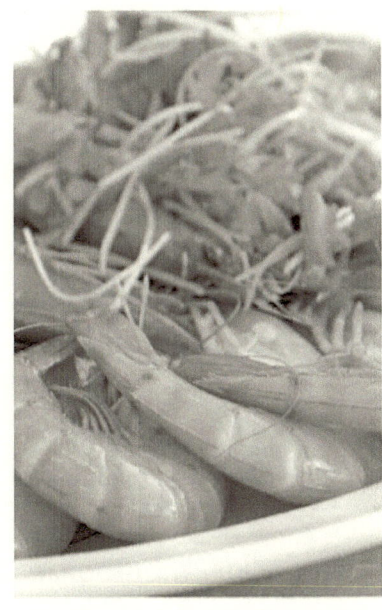

✓ Shrimp – 0 Carbs

✓ Crawfish - 0 Carbs

✓ Crab - 0 Carbs

✓ Lobster – 2 grams per 6 ounces

✓ Mussels – 8.4 per 6 ounces

✓ Oysters – 12.4 per 6 ounces

✓ Scallops – 3.9 per 6 ounces

✓ Clams – 8.7 grams per 6 ounces

✓ Squid – 7 grams per 6 ounces

Fats And Dressings

✓ Butter - 0 Carbs

✓ Mayonnaise - 0 Carbs

✓ Oils – 0 Carbs (olive, avocado, and coconut oils for general use. Cold-pressed or expeller-pressed canola, peanut, and grapeseed oils are good for stir-fries)

✓ Pure Unrefined Cold Pressed Extra Virgin Coconut Oil – 0 Carbs
(contains medium chain triglycerides fatty acids, metabolized by the body to be used as immediate energy and not stored as   fat)

✓ Blue Cheese Dressing (2 tbsp.) – 2.3 grams

✓ Italian Dressing (2 tbsp.) – 3 grams

✓ Cesar Dressing (2 tbsp.) - .5 grams

✓ Ranch Dressing (2 tbsp.) – 1.4 grams

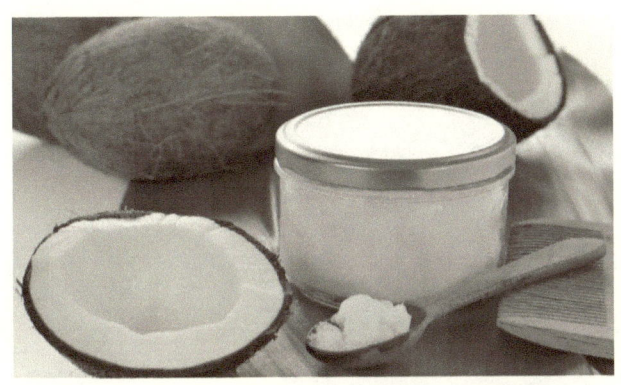

✓ 100 Island Dressing (2 tbsp.) – 4.8 grams

Note: Check labels on all commercial dressings for carb counts

Soy Vegan Protein

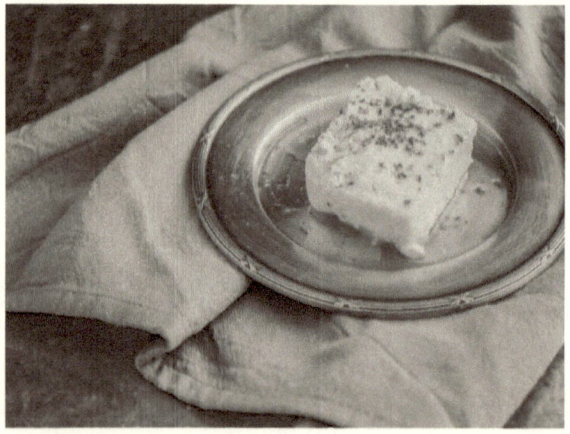

- ✓ Soybeans - 6.2 grams per 1/2 cup

- ✓ Soy Milk – 1.2 grams per cup

- ✓ Firm Tofu – 2.2 grams per 4 ounces

- ✓ Silken Tofu – 3.2 grams per 4 ounces

- ✓ Tempeh – 16 grams per cup

- ✓ Soy Nuts – 2 grams per ½ ounce

Vegetables

- ✓ Alfalfa Sprouts - .4 grams per cup

- ✓ Daikon – 1 gram per ½ cup

- ✓ Endive - >1 gram per ounce

- ✓ Escarole - >1 gram per ounce

- ✓ Arugula - .2 grams per ½ cup

- ✓ Bok Choy - .8 grams per 1 cup/raw

- ✓ Celery - .8 grams per 1 stalk

- ✓ Chicory Greens - .6 grams per ½ cup

- ✓ Green Onions - .1 per 1 tablespoon

- ✓ Cucumber - 1 gram per ½ cup sliced

- ✓ Fennel - 3.6 grams per 1 cup

- ✓ Iceberg Lettuce - .1 grams per 1/2 cup

- ✓ Jicama - 2.5 grams per ½ cup

- ✓ Parsley - >1 gram per ounce

- ✓ Bell Peppers - 2.3 grams per ½ cup

- ✓ Radicchio - .7 grams per ½ cup

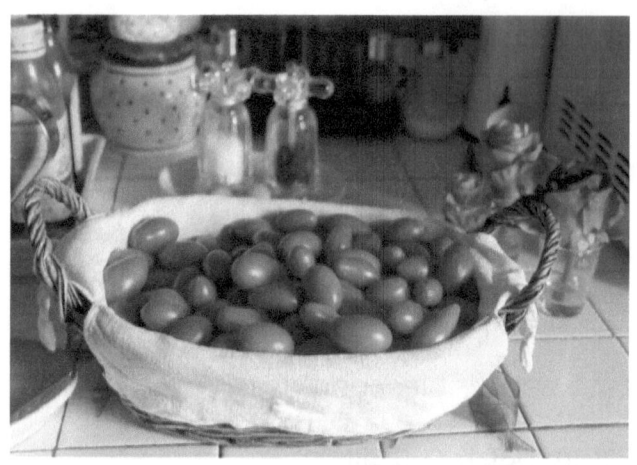

✓ Radishes - .9 grams per 10 pieces

✓ Romaine Lettuce - .2 grams per ½ cup

✓ Artichoke (1/4 Steamed) – 4 grams

✓ Artichoke Hearts In Water - 2 grams per 1 heart

✓ Asparagus - 2.4 grams per 6 spears

✓ Bamboo Shoots - 1.1 grams per 1 cup

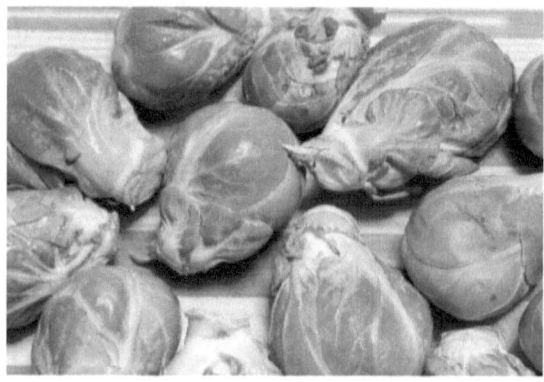

- ✓ Broccoli - 1 gram per 1/2 cup

- ✓ Brussels sprouts - 2.4 grams per ¼ cup

- ✓ Cabbage - 2 grams per ½ cup

- ✓ Cauliflower - 2 grams per 1 cup

- ✓ Chard - 1.8 grams per ½ cup

- ✓ Collard Greens - 4.2 grams per 1/2 cup

- ✓ Eggplant - 1.8 grams per ½ cup

- ✓ Hearts of Palm - .7 grams per 1 heart

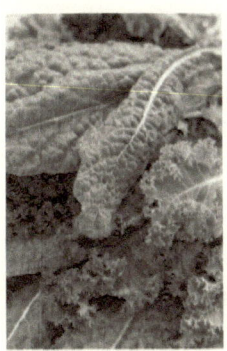

- ✓ Kale - 2.4 grams per ½ cup

- ✓ Mushrooms – 1 gram per ½ cup

- ✓ Kohlrabi - 4.6 grams per ½ cup

- ✓ Leeks - 1.7 grams per ¼ cup

- ✓ Okra - 2.4 grams per ½ cup

- ✓ Black Olives (10 small, 5 large, or 3 jumbo olives) - 1 gram

- ✓ Onions - 2.8 grams per ¼ cup
- ✓ Pumpkin - 2.4 grams per ¼ cup
- ✓ Sauerkraut - 1.2 grams per ½ cup
- ✓ Spinach - .2 grams per ½ cup
- ✓ Summer Squash - 2 grams per ½ cup
- ✓ Tomato (1 medium) - 4 grams
- ✓ Cherry Tomatoes - 4 grams per cup
- ✓ Turnips - 2.2 grams per ½ cup

Fruits

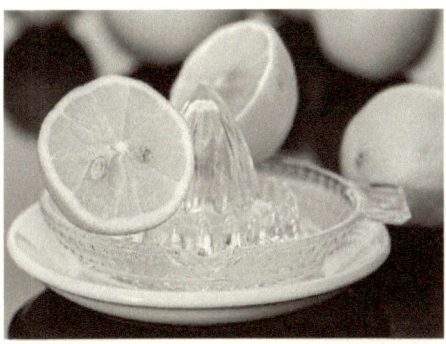

- ✓ Limes – 2 grams per 1 ounce
- ✓ Lemons – 2 grams per 1 ounce
- ✓ Rhubarb - 1.7 grams per ½ cup
- ✓ Avocado – 4.8 grams each
- ✓ Apricots – 5 grams per fruit
- ✓ Strawberries – 11 grams per cup
- ✓ Blackberries - 7 grams per cup
- ✓ Raspberries – 5 grams per cup
- ✓ Red Grapefruit - 9 grams per 1/2 fruit

Note: with the exception of lemons and limes in moderation, fruit is best introduced slowly into the diet once ketosis has been established and weight loss goals are being met, and you should monitor their effects on your weight loss and adjust as needed.

Dairy

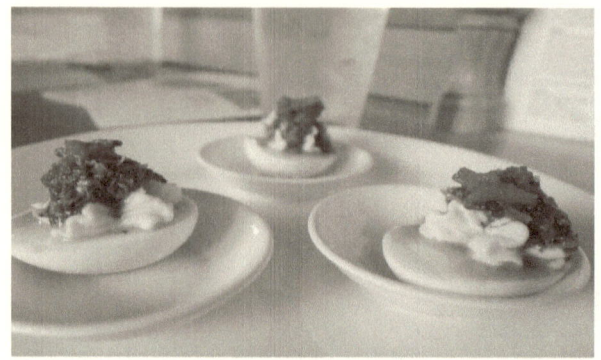

- ✓ Egg White – .3 grams

- ✓ Egg Yolk - .3 grams

- ✓ Whole Egg - .6 grams

- ✓ Heavy Whipping Cream - .5 grams per tablespoon

- ✓ Half-and-Half - .5 to 1 grams per tablespoon

- ✓ Plain Full Fat Greek Yogurt - 9 grams per cup

- ✓ Full Fat Sour Cream - 2 grams per 4 tablespoons

- ✓ Unsweetened Almond Milk – Less than 1 gram per cup

Cheeses

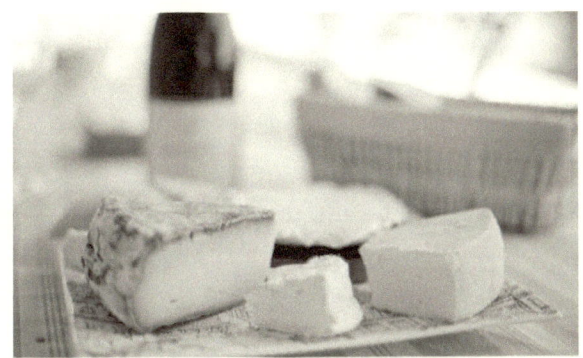

- ✓ Gruyère Cheese - .1 grams per 1 ounce

- ✓ Cheddar - .5 gram per ounce

- ✓ Fontina - .4 grams per 1 ounce

- ✓ Havarti - .7 grams per 1 ounce

- ✓ Parmesan - .9 grams per 1 ounce

- ✓ Gouda - .6 grams per 1 ounce

- ✓ Mozzarella - .6 grams per 1 ounce

- ✓ Ricotta - .8 grams per 1 ounce

- ✓ Blue Cheese - 1 gram per 1 ounce

- ✓ Edam - .4 grams per 1 ounce

- ✓ Monterey - .1 grams per 1 ounce

- ✓ Muenster - .3 grams per 1 ounce

- ✓ Provolone - .6 grams per 1 ounce
- ✓ Neufchatel - .1 to .8 grams per 1 ounce

Herbs And Spices

- ✓ All Herbs And Spices Have Very Few Carbs

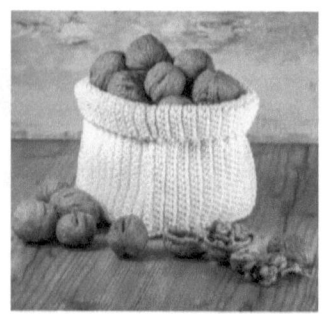

Nuts & Seeds

- ✓ Almonds (2 tbsp. whole) – 1.4 grams
- ✓ Peanuts (2 tbsp.) – 1.8 grams
- ✓ Hazelnuts (2 tbsp. chopped) - 1 gram
- ✓ Macadamia Nuts (2 tbsp. chopped) -.9 grams
- ✓ Pecans (2 tbsp. chopped) - .6 grams
- ✓ Pine Nuts (2 tbsp.) - 1.7 grams
- ✓ Pistachio Nuts (2 tbsp.) - 3.1 grams

✓ Walnuts (2 tbsp. chopped) - 1.1 grams

✓ Pumpkin Seeds - 5 grams per ounce

✓ Sunflower Seeds (2 tbsp.) – 1.5 grams

✓ Almond Butter - 3 grams per tablespoon

✓ Peanut Butter – 2.4 grams per tablespoon

Note: Like fruit, nuts are best introduced slowly into the diet once ketosis has been established and weight loss goals are being met, and you should monitor their effects on your weight loss and adjust as needed.

Zero Carb Drinks

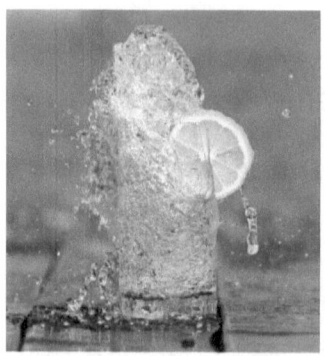

✓ Water

✓ Unsweetened Tea

✓ Unsweetened Coffee

✓ Club Soda

✓ Diet Soda (be cautious as artificial sweeteners

✓ can affect low carb weight loss)

✓ Sugar Free Sparkling Water

✓ No-Calorie Flavored Seltzers

✓ Herbal Tea (without added barley or fruit sugars)

Alcoholic Beverages

Pure Spirits Have 0 Carbs

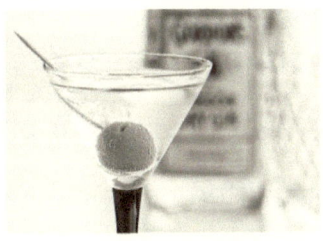

- ✓ Gin
- ✓ Rum
- ✓ Vodka
- ✓ Whiskey
- ✓ Martini
- ✓ Tequila

A small amount of alcohol typically will not disturb ketosis, but it has to be the right alcohol. This means no beer, which is basically liquid bread, and no sugary cocktails, such as Pina Coladas, Daiquiris, White Russians, or Margaritas.

Pure spirits are best and should only be mixed with sugar free liquids, like water, club soda or diet tonic. Wine, which has a low amount of carbs, is okay but in strict moderation.

Track your weight loss progress if you are drinking to see if the alcohol has any adverse effect on your weight loss, if your progress stalls eliminate liquor to see if that makes a difference.

Miscellaneous And Snacks

- ✓ Shirataki Noodles – 0 Carbs
- ✓ White Vinegar – 0 Carbs
- ✓ Balsamic Vinegar – 0 Carbs
- ✓ Red Wine Vinegar – 0 Carbs
- ✓ Rice Vinegar (seasoned) 3 grams per tbsp.
- ✓ Soy Sauce - 1 gram per tablespoon
- ✓ Mustard – 0 Carbs
- ✓ Unflavored, powdered gelatin (use as a binder in recipes) – 0 Carbs
- ✓ Most Hot Sauces – 0 Carbs
- ✓ Turkey or Beef Jerky (not teriyaki flavor) - 3 grams per ounce

- ✓ Kale Chips - 8 grams per ounce

- ✓ Coconut Flakes - 4 grams per ounce

- ✓ Pickles - 1 gram per pickle

- ✓ Pepperoni – check label for carb count

- ✓ Flaxseed crackers – check label, some brands have about 2 grams per cracker

High Carb Foods To Avoid

All Sugars

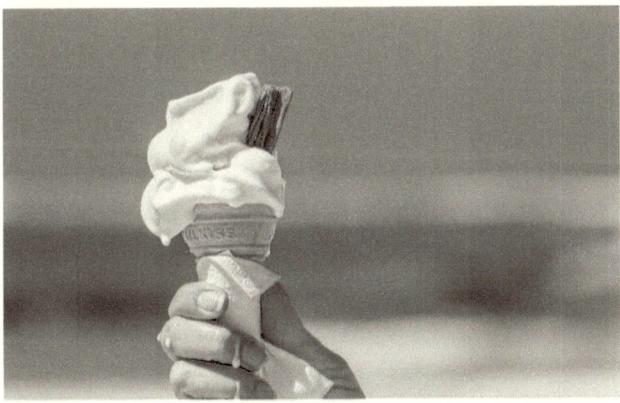

- ✓ White sugar

- ✓ Brown sugar

✓ Powdered sugar

✓ Any food with added sugar

✓ Processed food with added sugar

✓ Junk food with added sugar

✓ Jams and Preserves

✓ Some Sauces (check nutritional label and ingredients)

✓ Fructose (sugar in fruit)

✓ Some Salad Dressings (check nutritional label and ingredients)

✓ Cocoa mix

✓ Molasses

✓ Honey

✓ High-fructose corn syrup and foods made with it

✓ Syrups

Baked Goods and Sweets

✓ Cookies

✓ Cake

✓ Pie

✓ Brownies

- ✓ Donuts
- ✓ Pastries
- ✓ Muffins
- ✓ And all others

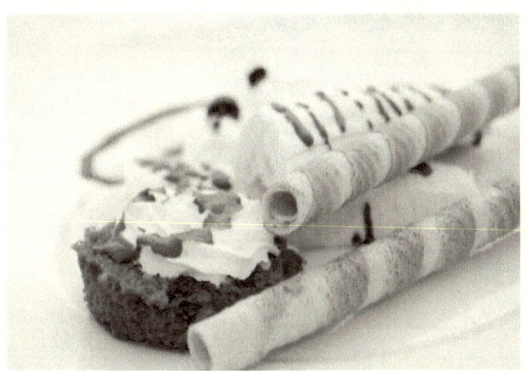

Candy

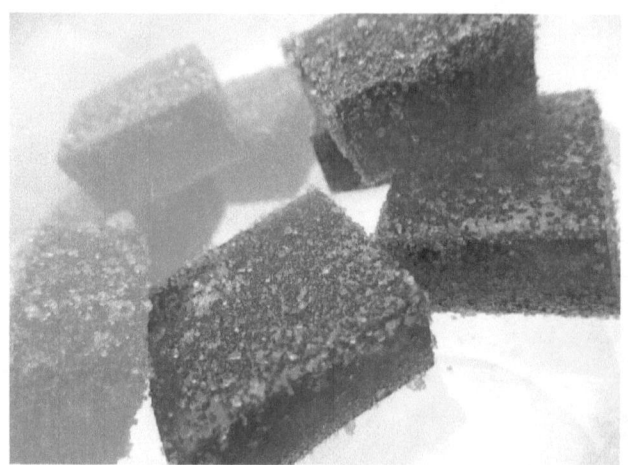

✓ Hard Candy

✓ Milk Chocolate

✓ Cotton Candy

✓ And all others made with sugar

✓ Chocolate Bars

Packaged/Processed Snacks

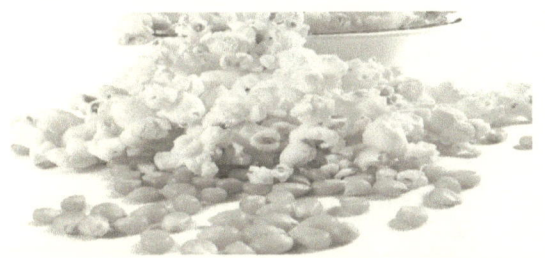

✓ Flavored Nuts

✓ Pretzels

✓ Rice Cakes

✓ Breakfast Bars

✓ Cheese and Crackers Snacks

✓ Raisins

✓ Potato Chips

✓ Tortilla Chips

✓ Popcorn

✓ Pop-tarts

✓ Granola Bars

✓ Twinkies

✓ Cupcakes

✓ And other boxed snacks and products

Dairy

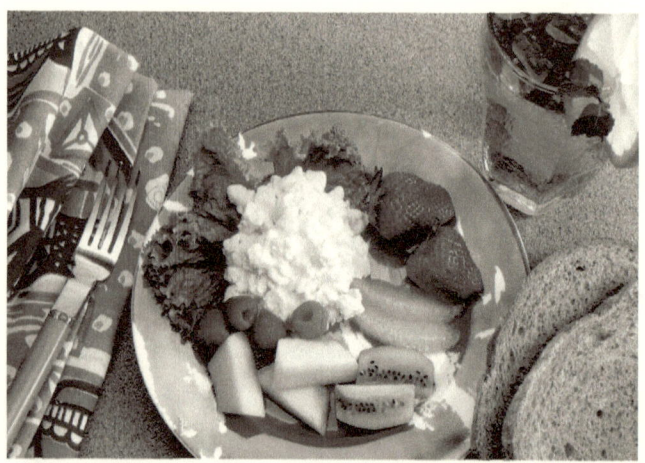

✓ Flavored Dairy

✓ Added Sugar Dairy

✓ Fruit At The Bottom or Sugar Added Yogurt

✓ Whole and Skim Milk

✓ Soy Milk

✓ Ice Cream

✓ Margarine

✓ Pudding

✓ Cottage Cheese

Sugary And Starchy Fruit

Medium Sugar Fruit

- ✓ Blueberries
- ✓ Coconut Meat
- ✓ Cantaloupes
- ✓ Watermelons
- ✓ Nectarines
- ✓ Papaya
- ✓ Peaches
- ✓ Apples
- ✓ Grapefruit
- ✓ Honeydew Melons
- ✓ Guavas
- ✓ Apricots

High Sugar Fruit

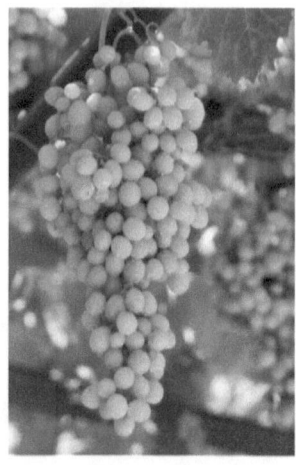

- Oranges

- Kiwifruit

- Pears

- Pineapple

- Plums

- Cherries

- Grapes

- Figs (Also Starchy)

- Bananas (Also Starchy)

- Mangos

- Tangerines

- Pomegranates

- Dates

- Applesauce

- Dried fruit (worst choice as it has very high concentrations of sugar from the drying process)

Starchy Vegetables

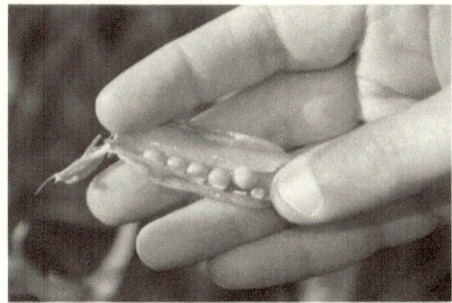

✓ White Potatoes (French fries and potato chips)

✓ Sweet Potatoes or Yams

✓ Corn

✓ Peas

✓ Squash

✓ Root vegetables not advised for very low carb diets (beets, carrots, parsnips, rutabaga, turnips, butternut squash, and winter squash)

Grains And Starches

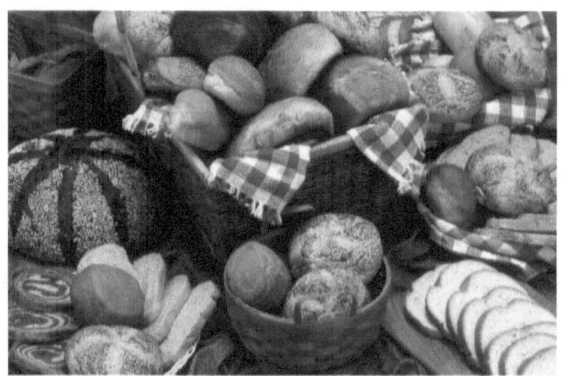

- ✓ Any Fried Food

- ✓ White Rice

- ✓ Bread, Bagels and English Muffins

- ✓ Croissants

- ✓ Tortillas

- ✓ Pasta

- ✓ Cold Breakfast Cereals

- ✓ Oatmeal

- ✓ Cream of Wheat

- ✓ Porridge

- ✓ Barley

- ✓ Amaranth
- ✓ Millet
- ✓ Quinoa
- ✓ Spelt
- ✓ Couscous
- ✓ Bulgur
- ✓ Rye
- ✓ Muesli
- ✓ Crackers
- ✓ Pizza
- ✓ Corn Starch
- ✓ Pancakes
- ✓ Waffles
- ✓ French Toast
- ✓ White Flour
- ✓ Whole-Wheat Flour
- ✓ Rice Flour
- ✓ Corn Flour
- ✓ All Whole Grains Too

Legumes

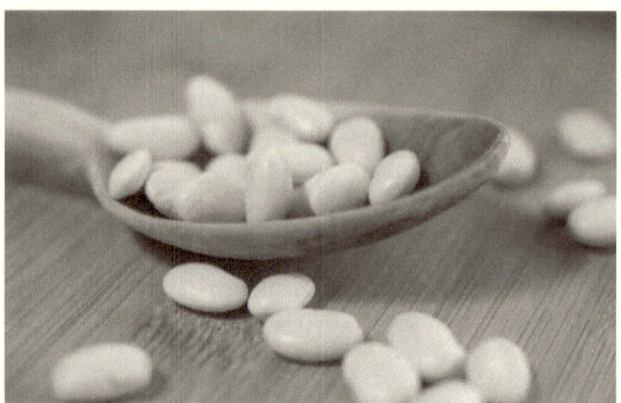

- ✓ Pinto Beans
- ✓ Black Beans
- ✓ Kidney Beans
- ✓ Chickpeas
- ✓ Navy Beans
- ✓ Lima Beans
- ✓ Baked Beans
- ✓ Lentils

Drinks

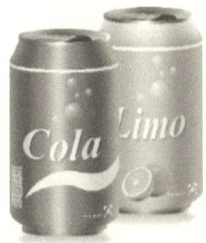

- ✓ Soda
- ✓ Juice
- ✓ All Sweetened Drinks
- ✓ Sweetened Or Flavored Tea
- ✓ Sweetened Or Flavored Coffee
- ✓ Frappuccino Coffee Drinks
- ✓ Milk Shakes
- ✓ Root Beer Floats
- ✓ Malts
- ✓ Frozen Coffee Drinks
- ✓ Sports Drinks (unless zero calorie)
- ✓ Beer

- ✓ Sweet cocktails – (Pina colada, daiquiri, mai tai, bloody Mary, margaritas, screwdriver, white Russian, rum drinks etc.)
- ✓ Wine coolers and alcopops

Sample 1 Day Keto Menu

Breakfast

Eggs cooked in butter
Bacon or sausage
Black coffee or with stevia or Splenda and heavy cream or tea

Snack

Turkey lettuce wraps with mayonnaise

Lunch

4 to 6 oz. steak with onions and mushrooms
Grilled kale with butter and garlic or raw kale with dressing or lettuce salad with dressing
Water, herbal tea, no calorie flavored seltzer, or coffee with stevia and heavy cream

Snack

½ avocado or 10 olives or 1 ounce of cheese with cucumber or celery slices

Dinner

4 to 6 oz. Grilled chicken
Vegetables (broccoli, asparagus, greens, green beans, or other low carb vegetables, your choice) with butter _or_ salad (lettuce, tomato, onion, cucumber, sprouts, bacon bits) with olive oil and vinegar or a creamy dressing
Water, herbal tea, or no calorie flavored seltzer

Snack

Hard-boiled egg with smoked salmon _or_ flaxseed crackers with salsa

Note: Portion sizes are not included because you eat to satisfaction, and portions will differ among individuals and men and women. Make sure to measure you vegetable and dairy intake to account for the daily carb intake limits.

Eating Out

Eating out on a keto diet is easy; the key is making proper choices.

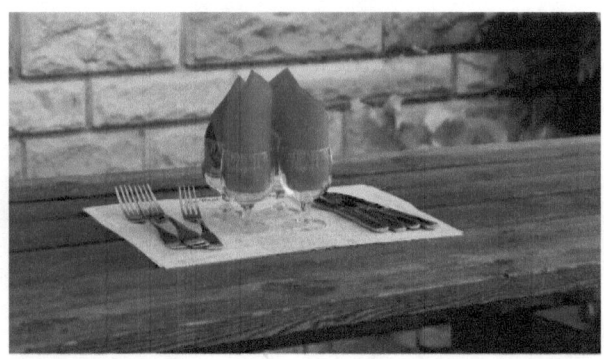

The main rules are:

- ✓ No starch

- ✓ No sugar

This leaves you with really unlimited possibilities for breakfast, lunch, and dinner.

Even fast food restaurants offer you low carb options, like getting your burgers lettuce wrapped, with a side salad instead of fries.

Mexican restaurants are okay too, just skip the chips, beans, and rice, and eat the meat and veggie fillings in burritos and tacos without the tortillas.

Italian places offer alternatives as well, where you can skip the bread and pasta, and eat pasta sauces over vegetables or chicken.

Carry a carb counter with you at all times so you can access the carb content of any food. These come in mini books or apps for your smartphones.

The main consideration when eating out is your own self-control, if you feel the temptation is too great, then avoid restaurants until you settle into your new low carb lifestyle and understand the best choices and swaps when eating low carb.

Testing For Ketones

There are various ketone-testing kits available, known as Ketosticks or Ketostix to test you urine for ketones. Your doctor can also order labs to test for ketones. This can be a good way to ascertain if your body has reached a state of ketosis and can be psychologically comforting. However, it is important to note that ketosis can be present without showing ketones in the urine.

Typically, a carb intake of up to 100 grams will induce ketosis, but ketones are rarely present in urine at this level of carbs in the diet.

Generally, ketones will show up in urine when intake is at 30 grams of carbs per day or less, though this too can vary.

One of the more important functions of ketone testing may be to allow the monitoring of the effects of carbs on ketosis as you progress. As you lose weight and progress towards your goal, you may begin to introduce more carbs to see the effect it has on your weight loss so you can find the right balance, and these test kits can be really helpful to that end.

Additionally, if you workout and as a result can tolerate more carbs and still lose weight, this testing may also help evaluate those efforts since as long as trace ketosis is maintained, carbs can be gradually added to the diet.

Results Will Vary

Some people can never seem to get past trace showings on the ketosis tests, while others consistently get darker readings, and there is little explanation for this.

It is best to not obsess about the results if you show lower than expected readings, and remember that just as finding dark readings can give you mental comfort, their absence can be distressing.

As long as you are losing weight, maintaining energy and feel good, that is all that matters.

Acetone Breath

Acetone breath or "keto breath" can indicate the presence of ketones, which turn to acetone in the body. The taste is typically metallic and easily fixed with sugar free gum.

Ketone Induced Changes In Urine

Ketosis can affect urine, creating a sort of distilled sour scent.

Optional Supplements

While no particular supplement is required, some can be very useful.

MCT Oil

Fatigue and weakness can occur when the body is not in full ketosis or is not fats and ketones efficiently. MCT (medium chain triglycerides) oil can help, as it provides energy and helps increase ketone levels. A couple of teaspoons of MCTs daily can help increase energy levels and decrease fat stores due to its thermogenic effect.

MCT's are found in coconut oil, but they are also offered in a purer supplement form called MCT oil that contains much more of the raw MCT's than coconut oil offers. It can be added to coffee, or mixed into dressings without any added taste.

Choose a quality MCT oil product that includes the highest level of caprylic acids, preferably pure, which act in the body as real MCT's and are able to bypass the metabolic burden of processing in the liver and quickly become energy in the muscles and the brain.

Caprylic acid has potent anti-microbial properties for healthy digestion and it only takes 3 steps to turn it into cellular fuel, versus sugar that takes 16 steps. It is highly ketogenic and quickly converts to ketones in the body.

This is especially useful in those with high levels of carb sensitivity, who have a hard time reaching high levels of ketones in their urine.

Caution: In some users, MCT oil can cause digestive problems and loose stools so it is best to start slow to allow the body to adjust, begin with a teaspoon at a time, and no more than 2 tablespoons a day and take it with food.

Consult your doctor before using, especially if you are prone to kidney stones.

Exogenous Ketones

This type of supplement can help raise the body's ketone levels and may be especially useful in those with high levels of carb sensitivity.

Whey Protein Shakes

Whey protein is a the highest quality protein supplement, and can help increase protein intake in a more convenient manner for those who lack it in their diet. Look for products with pure whey content, and not those that fluff their product with concentrates to get a more quality protein.

Multi Vitamin

Ask your doctor or nutritionist about taking a multivitamin that can boost nutrient intake.

Frequently Asked Questions

Q: How can it be healthy to cut out carbs from my diet?

A: The ketogenic diet does allow you to eat non-starchy vegetables, which are the healthiest carbs. It is the unhealthy carbs that are cut out, like refined sugar and sweets that do nothing but harm the body along with grains, like rice and pasta, and whole grains, which are counterproductive to weight loss and ketosis.

Another important factor is that while you eliminate carbs, you also increase intake of healthy fats and certain fats are very good for you, including avocado, meats, butter, cheese, coconut, and olive oil. Eating fat in the a low carb diet promotes fat burning, and remember many studies have shown that low carb diets are more effective than low fat diets in both weight lost and reducing heart disease risk factors.

Q: Won't the high fat intake cause high cholesterol?

A: Evidence suggests the opposite is true. Low carb eating has an edge over low-fat diets for improving good HDL cholesterol levels over the long term as shown by one of the longest studies done on the subject (but not the only one) and funded by the National Institutes of Health (published in the journal, Annals of Internal Medicine).

Q: Aren't whole grains good for me?

A: Whole grains are insulin triggers, and while they are often portrayed as healthy and necessary in a western diet, and that maybe true in some aspects, the fact is that whole grains often have a higher glycemic index than sugar itself. This means that eating raw sugar causes less of an insulin response in your body than a slice of bread. Many experts agree that humans can live without whole grains, and evolution apparently agreed, as early civilizations of man did not have access to grains and managed to thrive and survive.

Q: Are there any side effects to cutting out carbs?

A: Some people experience digestion and diarrhea problems, but this common side effect typically goes away after about four weeks. Eating more high-fiber vegetables, like leafy greens and broccoli helps and magnesium supplements can alleviate constipation.

Q: I only need to lose 20 pounds, is a keto diet for me?

Definitely, keto can help you lose 20 pounds or a 150 pounds. It can also help you gain more energy, and get control of your appetite.

Q: How long will it take to reach ketosis?

A: Ketosis begins when the glycogen in the liver is depleted. When you limit carbs to 50 net grams or less daily it typically takes no longer than 24 hours to enter ketosis.

Q: Is frequent urination normal?

A: Yes because the first two weeks of carb depletion is when a lot of water weight loss occurs as the liver begins to deplete its glycogen levels. Drink more water and pee on!

Q: Will I ever be able to eat pasta, bread or sugar again?

A: When following the Ketogenic diet it is very important to be strict in the elimination of carbs initially, to allow the body to fully enter ketosis. As you begin to lose weight, you can slowly integrate some carbs into your diet, typically in the form of more vegetables, nuts, and possibly berries. However, you need to monitor your weight loss to see how these carbs effect it, in order to find the right balance.

Once you reach your weight loss goals, you can indulge on occasion, but then return to the diet immediately. As with any healthy eating strategy, moderation is always key.

Keep in mind, keto is a lifestyle not a temporary diet, so you must be vigilant about your choices, basically forever, and returning to high carb eating will only lead to weight gain.

The common sense viewpoint is that whenever you return to a lifestyle that made you overweight to begin with, it can only do so again and again.

Q: How can I deal with missing sweets and carbs?

A: There is an adjustment period, and there may be struggles, but the truth is once you kick the sugar habit, your body and mind will adjust and you will be better for it.

Q: Is there a risk of muscle loss on low carb diets?

A: Many diets pose this risk, even the every day crappy eating that is so rampant in society with junk and processed food filling super market shelves. The high protein and ketone levels in a low carb diet help minimize muscle loss and it is always recommended to anyone to participate in regular strength training as part of an overall healthy lifestyle.

Final Thoughts

The best research in the world is your own, so get the go ahead from your doctor, and see for yourself if the Ketogenic diet can change your life.

A new body and far better health is waiting!

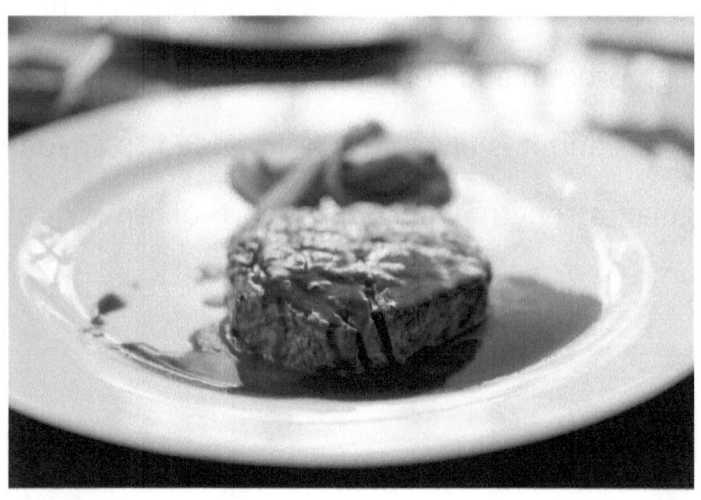